NATURAL HAIR CARE

The Easy Way

Kummbareh M. Owens

EverButter, LLC

Copyright Information

Copyright © 2018 by EverButter, LLC

Printed in the United States of America

First Edition

ISBN-13: 978-1985696648

Kummbareh Owens

EverButter, LLC

PO. Box 4294

Southfield, MI 48076

www.everbutter.com

Table of Contents

Preface

I am just going to stop you right there. If you want anything to become easy you have to forget what you thought you knew and relearn, retrain and rethink, put in some time. Then you form new thoughts, which forms new habits, which in turn will give you great ease. If you have bought this book, this means you want something that you are not getting from social media. So, get off. They are not your friends right now. It is time for you to go on a journey. I am glad you are taking me along that journey. It is time to rediscover who you originally been. Are you ready?

Throughout my 6 years of research into health and haircare, I have come to realize that all of our woes are a byproduct of what we do to our bodies. That includes what we eat by mouth and what our skin eats by application. When I started down this path, my daughter was having serious issues with her scalp. It was really concerning. Although her hair was growing it just wasn't vibrant and healthy looking. Her scalp was in very bad condition and the doctors didn't know why. I remember feeling bad because I would look at her scratch her scalp until it bled. Not only this I saw puss bumps and scaly patches on her scalp that made me want to cry. My daughter was in pain and I felt helpless. I assumed I was doing everything right, but little did I know, I was doing everything wrong.

Health for our child doesn't start when they are born. It starts with the mom, and the health of the mom's body before you even conceive. This is where I went wrong. During these years, although I didn't think I was eating bad, I was. I ate tons of processed foods; white flour, white sugar, table salt, packaged meats, cheese, desserts. Oh, how I loved desserts. I was eating how I was trained to eat. I thought what I ate was okay as long as it was in moderation. Although I did make sure I ate whole foods; vegetables, fruits they still weren't at the top of my list. I ate out with co-workers nearly twice a week. Went down to our bake shop for a snack nearly every day. This was my routine. I had no idea that what I was doing was not only hurting me but also my unborn children. "...most Americans now prefer to eat foods that we know shorten our lives and damage our brains. This damage also alters our genetic structure. Changes to our DNA accumulate from eating commercially designed foods that are incompatible with our genetic design. These gene defects have devastating consequences for us, but also can be passed on to our children and grandchildren." Fast Food Genocide

So, my daughter inherited a bad DNA structure from me, and we continued eating bad as I breastfed and as she gotten older. Which led to her diseased scalp. Doing my research, I stopped going to the doctor because they only prescribed these fake drugs that didn't help. I went over a course of 3 years and they had no clue on what to do. I was frustrated and tired. Upon doing research I quickly discovered that our products that we used every day was worsening the situation, and on top of that, the food she ate was horrible. You know as parents we think that snack food is a must. I kept crackers in our cabinet. The kids ate these all day every day. So, I did a clean sweep of all packaged foods. I stopped buying them, and then I started making her hair products. After making these small changes I saw some relief in her scalp. I had a long way to go but I was getting there.

6 years later our family is now completely plant based. Our goal was not to treat animals fairly, our goal is to be healthy. And being healthy means that we had to give up meat. My daughter is 7 now and I am still working with her and cleaning her system out. It is a little harder with her because she is so little. I can't do everything I do to myself, to her. They don't cooperate. They cannot suffer through drinking things that are not so pleasing and eating things that may taste horrible. But her scalp has made major improvements, regardless of the matter. I still have to stay on top of her eating habits. Retraining our kids mind has been so tough since we didn't start off this way. So, it has been a task to keep them away from households that does not share our same passion for health. Because I do notice when my daughter eats bad, she gets backed up fast and her scalp shows. I stay in their ears teaching them about the effects of food and how it plays a huge role in the quality of our life.

They don't understand completely but at least the conversation is being made.

Aside from my daughter having issues with her scalp, my two boys and girl were having teeth issues. Well, I should say my youngest boy and my girl started having cavities. This perplexed me so much. I was never the one to buy candy, chips and soda. We only drank water and candy was not allowed in the house. We did eat cakes, maybe once a week, but I didn't categorize that with candy. Come to find out is that all packaged foods contain high amounts of sugar; the white flour I was using, also sugar. And we consumed these things on a regular. So, although they didn't eat candy and drink pop, they were, because of the foods we ate. Over the course of 3 years we spent close to $4000 on their teeth. Ridiculous right? All avoidable if I stayed away from the American Standard diet.

It was our 5-year anniversary. We had already made plans to go to Puerto Rico. I had my yearly check up with my gynecologist. I go not thinking much of it. And she calmly tells me that she feels a lump on the side of my boob. She tells me not to worry that it may not be anything but she wants to be sure. She makes me an appointment to get an ultrasound. During that week I was freaking out. Who wants cancer? No one! I am calling everyone telling them to pray for me, because I need all that I can get. I go and he tells me it doesn't appear to be cancer, just a mass that is benign. Although I was relieved, I still wasn't. I knew that if I didn't change my lifestyle that that mass was going to come back and bite me. And so again, I began diving into research. Come to find out that everything from lotion to deodorant to hair products are dangerous. All of the commercial products lead to cancer or some other disease. And reading up on deodorant, I discovered that it was the most poison-ness thing we can apply to our body, especially antiperspirants. We are supposed to sweat, and when we don't, the toxins stay in our body causing bad problems. Sweat is just like pee and poop. You have to release the unwanted toxins, and if you don't poop or pee you end up having bladder infections and colon or intestinal problems. So just guess what happens if you don't sweat? I stopped wearing deodorant. It was a struggle because I was still eating toxic food. When you don't eat properly and you try to adopt a natural product lifestyle, they kind of work against each other. The natural deodorant wasn't really effective. You can't be natural in one thing and be unnatural in another, but I stayed with it. Once I went completely plant based, that is when I completely went off deodorant. I didn't have to wear it anymore. Surprisingly, I wasn't funky. I learned that our body does not put forth foul odors and if it does, it is coming from the toxic food and chemicals we are putting into our body and on our body. When I stopped eating processed foods my body started to operate properly. I still sweat a lot, but I am not funky...lol. What I didn't understand is that everything I was doing was going to cause me to have breast cancer. The products I put on my body and the food I ate. Eating processed foods, i.e. calorie rich and nutrient deficient; white flour, white salt, breads, pizza, pastries are high glycemic foods. These foods absorb rapidly in your bloodstream and causes so many ailments, which can be linked to, "colon cancer, breast cancer, endometrial cancer, lung cancer, pancreatic cancer and prostate cancer." Fast Food Genocide I was killing myself rapidly and didn't even know it. Whole and natural foods are made to digest slowly in our body. Nothing should digest quickly because one, you can't get all of the nutrients you are supposed to get from them. And 2, they go right into the bloodstream, go to the nervous system and really causes health issues that may happen now or happen later. Remember, there is always a cause to an effect. Nothing ever just happens. You may not be aware of the thing that happened, but it doesn't mean that there was something that caused it. If you have an ailment when you get older, diabetes, prostate cancer or whatever else, it is because of your eating habits and your parents habits and their parents habits. We don't get sick because we are old. We get sick because we have been putting the wrong thing into our body, and it finally caught up to us.

One more story. I have always had dandruff and in my early twenties I began suffering with acne. I had no idea these two were related until I started reading up on health. I went on for years assuming it was normal. My hair was growing but not as fast as it used to, and on top of that I had to cut my ends literally every month. We grow up knowing that we have to get our ends clipped every 6 weeks. This was normal behavior, so I didn't think much of it. I assumed the acne it was from stress. I started having acne when I entered college, so I linked it to that. I used all of the harsh facial stuff and it cleared up, but it came back after 6 months to a year. I would again use all of the harsh facial stuff and it would clear up, then when I hit about 33, it stopped clearing up. It started getting worse. I had ulcer like bumps in my cheek that would come every month, in which I blamed on my period. Those left dark marks every time. Then they started on my forehead, and it became a cycle. Nothing ever cleared it up fully. Years later I went plant based, and it was not because of acne or dandruff. It seemed to be logical due to my research. And crazy thing happened. I stopped getting dandruff and acne. My face is still going through detoxing and so I get minor breakouts but they don't linger around like it used to. As far as my dandruff, that has gone. And surprisingly enough I don't have to clip my ends so much. It's about twice a year now. In the winter, I do have to be careful cause dryness will dry your hair out too, so if I am not careful I will have to clip at least two times during the winter months if I am not moisturizing enough.

I say all of this because all of the things that were happening to me and my family was directly related to product usage, via food for the body or of the skin. What I will discuss in this book will make your hair care journey go a lot smoother and easier. What I say isn't rocket science, it's not even hard, it's straightforward and to the point. You may say to yourself, is this it? This is all I have to do? And the answer is yes. But the question is, will you?

Introduction

Natural hair is not about length, it's not about the perfect curl, it's not about flawlessness. I'm sorry to tell you, but social media is lying to you. They are selling you an image that is furthest from the truth. If you want your hair, your life to be easy, you have to become your own person. You have to get these images out of your head. You're going to have to kill the zombie inside of you. That seems like an oxymoron statement. How can you kill something that's already dead? But the zombie has been dead weight allowing you to behave in such a way that is not good for you.

This book is not going to be long and drawn out. It's going to be easy and to the point. They tell your life is hard, but it's not supposed to be. It should be easy. It's only hard when you're working outside of your genius. Basically, when you're trying to be something you're not.

At this point I probably should tell you who I am, but I'm not. It doesn't matter. All that matters is who you are, and who you plan to become.

Let's get started. With haircare and in life there are three major categories; Health, Regimen (process), and Dedication. Once you master these things, everything else will fall into place.

If you don't have good **health** you don't have anything. A lot of times we want to focus on the beauty aspect but not the actual thing that is the beauty. So, we focus on the face getting beat, and long hair and the bomb body, but eff all of them if your health is at risk. Other's hair can be long, and not trying to discredit them, but most of the time it is their genes that allows their hair to grow fast. Or they may be putting in a lot of work helping it to grow. Or, they could be young and vibrant and that's what youth do, everything grows fast. I say all of this because long hair doesn't mean anything, the best job ever or the biggest house or whatever you put at high esteem means nothing if you are not around to enjoy it. Long hair doesn't mean health, and short hair doesn't either, but if we can focus on health I can guarantee that length will follow. Maybe it will take longer than the next but that isn't the goal. The goal is making sure the inside of your body is functioning at its max.

With life you need a **regimen** to keep you on track. Things that you know will work every time and so you stick with it because it gives good results. To me that is the nature part of life. Nature will always act the same and give the same results. You can't go outside of nature and if you do, it will yield unpleasing results.

If you are not **dedicated** on improving, on achieving your goals, on making your life better, then you may as well give up now. This is why New Year resolutions fail, because they are made haphazardly, with no real truth behind them. You do it because it sounds good, because everyone else is doing it, but you didn't think about it, write it down, what it actually takes to achieve it. You didn't do anything. This is where dedication comes in at. Once you realize who you are and how you will become that best version, you have just dedicated yourself to only making goals that are in line with becoming your best self. You aren't too concerned with how others are living, with what others are saying, with how others are looking. You are dedicated to you. You are now writing down goals and not waiting until the New Year to be a new you. You are starting now. So, let's dedicate ourselves to becoming our best version now.

Health: Your Health Means Everything to Your Hair

-Buddha

In order for any of this to work, you have to start with your body. I think about Steve Jobs, he was at the epitome of his success. Brought life back to Apple, and then he ended up dying. He wasn't an old guy, 56. He easily could have had 30 more years left and even more but he fell ill and couldn't enjoy what he worked so hard to achieve. Which to me, is kind of a failure. You work so hard for something and then you can't even enjoy it. Health is one of those things that no one really ever talks about until some it sick or dying, but it has everything to do with everything. If you want to really enjoy your kids, you need good health. If you want to travel, you need good health. If you want to run a successful business, you need good health. If you just want to live an abundant life, you need good health. Sure, you can do all of these things and be in bad health, but you certainly will not enjoy them. When you feel horrible, life becomes a burden and you end up just wanting to die. Which is death, in essence. You are dead, but still breathing. Health is directly related to what we put into our bodies. If you have good health, you are putting good things in your body, i.e. whole foods, unprocessed and vice versa. Putting processed foods in your body will ultimately lead to dis-ease and then premature death. Constantly feeding our body with junk, highly chemical food will lead to "the destruction of human potential, along with the explosion of chronic illness, human suffering, and the premature death of millions." Fast Food Genocide. We cannot reach our highest potential while giving our body the lowest grade of food. Our brain cannot perform at its max, and neither can our body.

Let's talk about how health affects the hair. When your body is in a state of dis-ease, your head/hair will be one of the first indicators. Your head, hands and feet are your indicators to good health. These are the outputs of whatever you put into your body. Of course, we don't pay attention to the tale tell signs, but they are there. Things you will experience from the hair comes in the form of split ends excessively, dry hair, stagnant hair growth, dandruff (which includes (eczema, psoriasis, alopecia...etc.) these are pretty much all the same. Areas in your body, your organs, are not performing as they should and so one of these things arises. We assume all of these things are natural or out of our control or we think a product will solve the issue, but what a product does, is put a band aid on it and later it will come back with vengeance. Which is what medicine does, unless your medicine is food.

The first thing you want to do when starting this hair journey is to give your body a good cleaning. A lot of our issues come from a dirty colon and a dirty colon is because of a dirty liver. Liver is the central organ. It cleans the system. If it's junky, it cannot do its job properly, which means your other organs cannot do its job properly. Everything in our body is connected. You can't diagnose one thing without diagnosing the other. In our culture we are so used to healing the effect, but not the cause. I have this stomach ache and so we take antacids or what not to get rid of the ache, but we don't understand why it even happened in the first place. What was the cause of it? I have dandruff, and so we go to the store to get some head and shoulders. Well, that is only a temporary fix, because you are not fixing what is causing the dandruff?

Once we figure out the causes that is when a product can work it's best. A product, such as a haircare product can only enhance what you have. It cannot give you something you don't. One will keep going from product to product hoping it will fix their issues when what they are really looking for is a diet change. To begin healing oneself inside, so that the outside can reflect that.

Our head can be divided into sections. Each section is connected to an organ. Let's say you keep having dandruff in the crown of your head, you can pinpoint the organ in which it is connected to and understand that this organ is not running properly. What are the steps I need to follow in order to heal it? "The hair color, split ends, length of hair, texture and falling out of hair, along with the condition of the scalp; oiliness and dryness of the hair, and how slowly or quickly the hair grows in areas, indicates deterioration of health or dis-ease of specific organs. Hair represents all the body and all the body represents the hair." Dr. Llaila O. Afrika, African Holistic Health

Here I want to show you each section and what organ it is related to. When I came across this, I thought I hit gold...lol, but in the book African Holistic Health I found a diagram and I think it is something we all can benefit from. Now, it has an actual picture but I will explain in words each section. The book I am referencing is not about hair, but it gives some insight on it. In case you want it buy it, it is about health in general.

Front of head (hairline) - Excretory system, kidney, bladder, sex organs

Side of head - Lungs, large intestines, respiratory system

Top of head (crown) - Blood, circulatory system, small intestines, heart

Towards back side of head - Digestive system, stomach, side pancreas, spleen

Back near neck - Liver, gallbladder

Found in *African Holistic Health* book.

If you are ready to get serious about your hair, the first place to start is inside of your body. What is inside will reflect outside. Here are some suggestions on how to get started.

You would want to begin cleaning out your intestines and colon. If you have a dirty colon than your scalp definitely is at risk and your hair can't thrive as it should. The thing with having anyone of these organs not functioning right leads to the others not functioning right which leads to us not being able to absorb all of the nutrients that we need from food because our organs (kidneys, liver, gallbladder, stomach, intestines) is not running properly. It only makes sense to clean out the bad stuff we put in so we can start new.

Cleanses and Detoxes:

Cascara Sagrada

This is an all-natural herb that will get inside of the intestinal wall and clean you out. It's also a natural laxative which will help you get regular if you are not. I wouldn't start off so aggressive with cleaning, and this herb is gentle if used properly.

- I started Cascara Sagrada in the beginning of my journey. It is only recommended to do it no more than 1-2 weeks. That is what it takes, and it helps right away. If I go out of town I will take a teaspoon of this the first day back to cleanse myself out. When you are on vacation and you eat out every day it is important to detox when coming back.

Detoxes

Fruit, water, herbal teas, juice detox are always good ones. Some do them for a week or just a few days at a time, building themselves up to a week. Detoxing helps to rid the body of toxins from your organs and blood. A lot of people have unnatural ways to detox, but stick with the natural remedies. Doing a detox once a month is a good habit.

- I do a fruit detox in the warmer months when we get the sun in abundance once a month. I only do it for 2 days each month but I do this to give my body a break and to flush out all the bad stuff. I don't detox in the winter because of the sun exposure is minimal. I feel like I need all of the nutrition I can get in the winter months.

Whole Psyllium Husk

Taking a tablespoon of this every morning will help to clean the colon. This is high in fiber and is able to really get into the walls of the colon.

- Of course, I didn't take this while I did the cascara Sagrada, that would be bad. I started this midway into my plant-based journey, the first year. I took a tablespoon of it blended with strawberries mixed with 8 ounces of water every day for about 4 months. I felt like it was time to stop after that.

Salt Flush

You would take 1 tablespoon of natural salt, pink salt or Epsom salt and mix it with 16 ounces of water. Drink this after you drank at least 8 ounces of water in the morning. A salt flush is a laxative and cleanse.

- It made me sick for about 10-15 minutes where I had to sit down and close my eyes and then I had to eliminate and I felt so much better. It did what it was supposed to do. It pulled out all of the toxins which made me sick for a minute and then allowed me to eliminate. I only did this one time. I was so nervous about putting that much salt in my body, but I had no adverse effects. I used pink salt.

Colonic

This is something you may not want to do, but it does get a lot of junk that has been in your system for decades out. Men have been threatened as of late to get colon cancer and prostate cancer. It's all due to have a junky colon. So, clean your colon out. Research it and see if it is for you.

- After I did the kidney cleanse, and liver cleanse I went on and did a colonic. The place I went to was decent enough. My experience was discomfort, but I think it was due to the fact that I went 1 day after I did the liver flush. I was still gassy from that. So, I think it was a bit much for my body. I went again a week later and it was much better. They recommended that you get a colonic once a year. I am not sure if I will go that often but I will definitely do it more.

Kidney Cleanse

Kidney failure has become very common. It is common because all of the junk we put into our body, processed foods, pop, and alcohol. It is good to do a thorough kidney cleanse to help gently remove stones. I drink an herbal tea to specifically help with this, and here is the recipe.

- 1 oz marjoram

- 1 oz cat's claw

- 1 oz comfrey root

- 2 oz fennel seeds

- 2 oz chicory root

- 2 oz uva ursi

- 2 oz hydrangea root

- 2 oz gravel root

- 2 oz marshmallow root

- 2 oz goldenrod herb

(Recipe found in "The Amazing Liver and Gallbladder Flush")

If you cannot find all of them, no worries, just mix what you have. But I did go on www.mountainroseherb.com to order all of mine. Make 8 ounces a day for 21 days and drink it throughout the morning. You don't want to gulp it down. Allow it to get into your system gently and smooth. This helps to clean out your intestines as well.

- This was a non-eventful cleanse but you can tell that it was cleaning you out. But it is very gentle and no bother. You do feel lower back pain for about a day, but that means that the stones are moving out, which is a good thing.

Liver Cleanse

A liver cleanse is the last step to cleaning out your entire system. This is what you have been prepping for. There are several different ways you can do one and it's detailed. I would suggest you researching it on your own to see exactly what it is all about. Then you can see if it is something you want to do. A good resource for this information is "The Amazing Liver and Gallbladder Flush" by Andreas Moritz

- I didn't enjoy doing this because it's a lot of little things you have to do. And the drinks were not as tasty, but I got through it. It is recommended to do these for as long as it takes to get all of the stones out. You actually get to see the stones coming out.

Note - Avoid doing any cleanses and flushes if you are pregnant, or have a major illness. I am no doctor, I have just researched and have performed these cleanses on myself. And they have changed my health for the better.

Please do the research for yourself to determine if these cleanses are for you.

One more thing I would like to mention concerning your health is exposure to the sun. Our livelihood comes from the sun. We would not be able to live and survive. The sun is much needed for the health of our body which includes our scalp and skin. When we do not allow our scalp to be exposed to the sun due to us wearing wigs or sew ins, we are not allowing the nutrients from the sun to get absorbed into our scalp leaving our scalp and hair damaged. We have to allow our scalp to breath and have fresh air, and exposure to the sun. If we do not, our hair will become very weak and growth will be nonexistent. Our hair health is determined from our scalp health. The sun heals, kills germs and diseases and gives nutrients, so allow the sun to do what it is supposed to do. One would never want to use sun block. The sun is not what we should be afraid of, it's the food we eat on a regular, that we should be most afraid of.

You have done all the cleanses but how do you go about eating and purging your cabinets? That is pretty easy. If you are new to this healthy way of eating, you have been following the American standard diet, then throw out all processed foods. That means all of your frozen pizzas, waffles, fries, ice cream. All of the things you just need to pop in the oven for a bit and eat. Then go to your cabinets and throw out all of your snacks; chips (even tortilla), cookies, juice boxes, crackers, basically anything in a box that last a long time on the shelf. Your next thing is to go shopping for whole foods; veggies, fruits, nuts, beans, lentils, all things that are high nutrient and low in calories. We want nutrient dense foods, not calorie rich. One thing is to prepare all of your food at home, eat as much raw foods as possible; salads, fruits and nuts.

There is an elephant in the room. Do you have to go plant based? Yes, wholeheartedly. This is not something I can say is a choice thing or depends on who you are. Nope, everyone needs to go on a plant-based nutrition diet, but going plant based is not something that is that easy to do. We have trained ourselves to think one way and now the un programming has to start and that is a process. Basically, going plant based is something you have to come to the conclusion of on your own. If you do it and not mean it, you will go right back to your old ways. I researched for nearly a year and at the end of that research I went cold turkey cause the evidence was undeniable. What I would recommend to you is to invest in discovering as much as you can about health and the way food impact that, and then come back to the question, should I go plant based? Purchase the books I mentioned in here, that's a good starting point. Because making the decision you have to be firm in it because people will laugh at you, criticize you and just make you feel as if it's the worst thing you could do. You will have to sit there and watch others eat because the majority of people are not plant based. You will have to prep all of your food, snacks and lunches cause eating out is not an option for you anymore, because you choose health over convenience. It's not going to be easy and simple, due to the way our society is set up. So, when you go plant based, you have to mean it.

Example, my husband decided to go plant based after about 3 months of me transitioning. When he first went he was all in. If we went to a restaurant he would stick as close to vegan as possible. He embraced all of the food I cooked and loved it. Then, he slowly but surely started to fade. Although I didn't cook him anything other than vegan, he stopped and got his junk when he wanted. He finally changed back but this time he wasn't doing it off of what I told him. He actually did a little reading and research. After that he was convinced that plant based was the only logical thing. Like I said, it is better that you research and see for yourself. We were taught at a very young age to just believe what I say and don't research anything. Now we are at a point where information is free flowing. Anything you want to know is at your fingertips, so go out and discover for yourself. Allow this book to be your stepping stone.

While you are researching I would recommend that if you can't stop eating meat right away, start by taking meat out of one of your meal times. Ease yourself into cutting out meat all together. Stop eating meat with breakfast, once you are used to that, stop eating it during lunch. Then dinner. Then maybe you can make a goal to only eating it over the weekend. Finding recipes is easy. Go on YouTube and look up some of your favorite meat meals, but vegan. Search, vegan tacos. You will get a slew of things that come up. Search healthy vegan snacks. This can start you off. And once you are fully committed, you will figure it out from there. The universe will give you all that you need at the time you need it.

>>> If you would like more information on developing your moisture regimen that works for you sign up for our FREE Moisture Regimen Hacking Course at:

www. everbutter.com/MRH

Regimen: The Process to Perfection

Sometimes we make the process more complicated than we need to. We will never make a journey of a thousand miles by fretting about how long it will take or how hard it will be. We make the journey by taking each day step by step and then repeating it again and again until we reach our destination.

-Joseph B. Wirthlin

It's all in the regimen. Once you figure out what works and you continue to do it, it becomes habit, and that is what you want. In order to establish a good hair habit, is by first finding out what products your hair likes and then following a good healthy regimen.

When you transition, big chop, and then growing the hair out, you actually can find yourself changing products for each stage. Although you may be using different products, the regimen will stay the same. So, focus more so on the regimen in the beginning and not the products. Then once you find your groove you will be finding yourself eliminating products you don't like and what you do. You may add things here and there, as your hair grows out or even delete things, but the key is in the regimen. I go in depth on this topic in our free online course, Moisture Regimen Hacking - 6 Steps to Get Your

Moisture Regimen Together which you can find at everbutter.com/MRH. It will give you tons of information that I don't mention in here.

What does a good regimen consist of you ask?

Properly following a moisture routine during the week. This is your maintenance routine, mostly it will be done at night. Take your hair down, moisturize it, secure it in a no tension style, i.e. twist, braids, bun and apply a satin/silk hair scarf. Moisturizing your hair throughout the week is critical. Especially during the winter months. Textured hair dries out fast, due to the curls. I get a lot of questions with people asking how often to moisturize. Ladies think a product is not working because they say they have to use it every day. For the most part, in your early stages when you are going on this health journey, you will have to apply every day. As your body gets healthier, and you're following a good regimen, you will find where it may be every other or maybe just once during the week, but I don't recommend going more than two days without moisturizing.

Your moisture routine will also include a step by step wash day. Where you are pre-treating the hair, cleanse with a gentle cleanser, deep condition, use a leave in, moisturizer and sealer. It's nothing to this, it's just following it to a T. At least in the beginning so that your hair will get to healthy. Once your hair is healthy, you can ease up. Meaning that if you are in a rush you may can skip pre-treating and deep conditioning, but it's not an all the time thing. You still want to practice good habits but if you miss a week in doing it step by step it will not hurt you.

Wash day regimen

Pre-treatment

Pretreatment is when you condition the hair before washing the hair. This may seem backwards but the reason behind this is that it detangles and moisturize the hair before opening the hair cuticle with a cleanser so that you will only clean always the dirt and grime without losing your natural oils. And by detangling it beforehand helps the hair not be so tangled after washing. Wetting the hair when you have not gotten the loose and shedded hair out gets tangled in and makes it that much harder to detangle afterwards.

Cleanse

You should use a very gentle cleanser. A cleanser can dry the scalp and hair out if it's not a natural one. The proper technique in cleansing the hair is to apply the cleanser directly to scalp and gently scrub. You will then rinse gently allowing the suds to run down the length of the hair to get access dirt and grime. You do not want to apply the cleanser directly to hair unless you are clarifying the hair which should take place once a month.

Deep Condition

A deep conditioner is critical in the process. This is the only product that will get inside of the hair cuticle to repair and strengthen. This sets the tone of how well your hair will be moisturized throughout the week. A good deep conditioner is that which has herbs/botanicals, protein with good humectants, and good butters and oils. If it does not have protein in it, that is fine, but you do want to use one at least twice a month.

Leave-in

A leave in helps the hair retain moisture. A leave in is recommended so that your hair is balanced.

Moisturizer

A moisturizer should be used right after a leave in. It helps seal in everything you just did to it and keeps your hair moisturized and strong. A moisturizer is most of the time the style.

Sealer

Sealing in the moisture rather you have high or low porosity is critical. It prevents the hair from drying out so fast. This can be a butter or oil.

Weekly regimen

- This is pretty simple. After each night, pull your hair down; section in 4, apply a spray moisturizer or water, then apply a sealer, either a butter or oil and twist, braid or bun the hair. Always apply a satin or silk scarf. The braids or twist can be as large as you want. If you are going for a twist, medium size is usually good.

There are other elements in why your hair may need more moisture and when to know when it is the product not moisturizing enough and not your hair.

Porosity

Porosity is the level at which your hair can receive moisture. Some have harder times than others and this is where the problem lies. There are 2 porosity levels that needs to be mentioned. High and low porosity.

Low Porosity

Low porosity is when the hair cuticle, which is the outer layer of the hair shaft lays flat. Think about the stem of a flower, it is sleek, not much water will penetrate. People with low porosity will have a difficult time choosing products that will not sit on top of the hair but will penetrate. Heavier products may tend to weigh the hair down. Depending on the person, one may like this, but some do not. With low porosity it is not a question on if moisture will penetrate, it will. It is a question on how long it will take to penetrate. Just know that you may need a full 2 days before taking down twist or braids. Things that will help with moisture retention are higher pH products which are usually, leave ins, high in humectants, and water-based products. Using protein when you are not moisturizing regularly will cause the hair to get dry and brittle. When using protein on low porous hair one must make sure to be using high moisturizing products.

High Porosity

This is when the hair cuticle is open. If you have high porosity you may experience moisture leaving your hair within a half hour to an hour after putting it in. It feels good going on, but it never stays that way. Products you should gravitate to are high emollient products. Heavier oils and butters. You should also practice the L.O.C method. Which should be done each time you moisturize and wash the hair. (L - Leave in, O - Oil, C - Cream, moisturizer) One would want to apply each product after the other when performing the LOC method. Making sure to use protein very often is needed. You should be using a conditioner with protein in it every week and use a style that has protein.

To determine your level

Step 1 - Grab a cup of water

Step 2 - Take clean hair from your comb after it has been washed. Or you can clip a few strands.

Step 3 - Place hair gently into the cup. Make sure not to force the hair to go down.

Step 4 - Observe to see if hair falls to the bottom or stay at the top.

Step 5 - If it sinks to the bottom you have high porosity

Step 6 - If it floats on the surface of the water, you have low porosity

Step 7 - If it sinks to the middle, your hair is medium porosity which is average/normal.

Or you can take our Hair Porosity Quiz at everbutter.com/pq

Things that can alter your results is having product on the strands when doing it. If you do have product on the hair, it will sink to the bottom. But after 10 minutes the product will come off and it will either stay at the bottom or rise to the middle or top showing its true porosity level.

Also note that the health of your hair will determine how difficult it is to moisturize the hair. High porosity and low porosity hair will not be a big issue if you take care of your hair, treat it well and put the proper things into your body. Your products will work better and your hair will accept it better.

Climate change

When it begins to get cooler, one would want to change to styling products that do not contain humectants. Why? Humectants, i.e. honey, vegetable glycerin, aloe gel, etc. draws moisture to them. Which is amazing in the summer, because it is a lot of moisture in the air. But when it is cold outside, and it is not that much moisture in the air, these humectants leave the hair in attempt to find like molecules. Which means it takes moisture out rather than putting it in. This is when it is the products fault, and not your hair. Change your products the same time you start changing the clothes you wear.

This concludes how a good regimen should be started. You cannot go wrong with this method. You can add to or delete as time goes by.

Note - using protein is beneficial for all hair types. Using a deep conditioner with protein in it weekly or biweekly will be enough.

>>> If you would like more information on developing your moisture regimen that works for you sign up for our FREE Moisture Regimen Hacking Course at:

www. everbutter.com/MRH

Dedication: The Engine to Success

If you believe in yourself and have dedication and pride - and never quit, you'll be a winner. The price of victory is high but so are the rewards.

- Paul Bryant

Dedication - *"to devote wholly and earnestly, as to some person or purpose"* Dictionary.com This definition speaks to me and tells me that in order to accomplish anything, you have to put your whole heart into it. Meaning, patience, diligence and sacrifice. There is no other way.

I remember drifting along, not having a clear direction, path or purpose. I hated where I was at, but had no clue in how to get to where I wanted. I was frustrated, and mad at the world. I wasn't happy for anyone and their good fortune, because I was lost in my own misery. I had completely given up on me. I dedicated my whole life to pleasing others and that got me know where. I dedicated my life to being this ideal person, that I thought could propel me into greatness. Ultimately, I was dedicating my life to misery. There is that dedication, but it was directed in the wrong thing. At the time, I didn't look at it as me dedicating myself to these things, but the definition says "wholly" to a person or purpose. For the longest I thought my purpose was to be nice, do as I was supposed to, and everything else will fall into place, but I was miserable. Be careful in what you dedicate yourself to.

In an attempt to find myself, my life's purpose, I had an epiphany. I was going to blog. I loved writing and I loved hair, and so that was what I was going to do. I had my husband set me up a site and I wrote my first blog. That first blog went nowhere. I was disappointed because no one read it, I got no likes and so I quit. I didn't go back to write another one, but here I am, having wrote 2 books and this will be my third book, with tons of blogs and hair tips under my belt. Why did I quit then and not now? It's not because I am getting tons of attention, likes and accolades. Nope. It is definitely dedication. During that time, I saw where people were getting tons of praise for their blogs and having tons of success, and I wanted that. I wanted to be somebody. I didn't sit down to think about my goal and a game plan. I didn't make a success plan; which was my end goal. All I wanted was fame, which is why it ended so soon. I wasn't dedicated to the mission. I wasn't dedicated at all, but now being in a better mental state I know exactly what I want to achieve. I have written down my mission statement, wrote out my vision and plans. I know exactly my end goal, which isn't fame, if I may add. Dedication is allowing me to stay in it until I win it. I am not going to give up because of the non-likes or accolades. I have put in a lot of work beforehand to get to where I am now, so now I am at the point of no return. That is dedication my friends. Getting to a point where you can't give up even if you wanted to, because the pre-work has been so much.

Dedication is that one thing that you need in order to get anything done. To change old habits. To keep that new year's resolutions. To build a successful business, and without saying, to have healthy hair. If you cannot commit and dedicate the time needed to get to your goal in your natural hair journey, you have already failed. This part of your journey should be personal. Getting to know your hair is a spiritual journey, because you are not just getting to know your hair, but getting to know your body, getting to know you. On this journey you will have so many emotions, but it is worth it. Keeping your eye on the prize is difficult when you see the ending of your destination. Seeing someone on IG, Facebook, or YouTube with their glorious hair, or life. Your kind of instantly feel defeated. Thinking that it is taking too long for your hair to grow, or your curls aren't cute because it doesn't look like their curls. Or you may not get as many likes as the next person gets. All of this is illusion tactics to get you off your grind. Get off of social media and focus on you. Get your mind, body and spirit in line. Once you have achieved that, then get back on if that's something you want to do. But you may say, "nah, I'm good."

Dedication can mean cutting things off, losing friends, family, material assets on the journey. Are you prepared for that? When you are dedicated, you allow the universe to do what is needed so that you can become your best version of yourself.

As I became more dedicated into becoming my best version, I saw myself being more intolerable of how people treated me, how and what they say to me. I started wanting to know more and more information, and so I began reading more, started journaling more, writing down my visions more. I got off of social media and stopped liking the things that I thought gave me pleasure and joy. I started to become more at peace with being alone. During this transformation, I was not expecting or even aware of the death blow that was going to occur.

I am from a family of 13, I have 7 brothers and 5 sisters. We were raised very close, talk and see each other on a regular. Well as any normal day, one day out the blue, several of them decided they didn't like who I was becoming. They didn't like my expansion of my thoughts. My wanting to learn more and questioning everything. It began with me not being able to come to their home, and after that, I took it from there. I totally blocked them from my life; blocked numbers, deleted Facebook accounts, unfollowed, I did everything. And funny thing is that if they would have done that to me several years back I probably would have lost it. But the new me, I allowed myself to grieve over it, to be upset, but I gave myself a week, and then I moved on. I love my family no doubt, but I am dedicated to my mission and will not allow anyone to disrupt in who I am becoming. I am a caterpillar right now, and I am preparing to become a beautiful butterfly.

As I went cold turkey into plant-based diet I had no clue how that would affect my social life. I didn't really consider others when I made my decision, as the way it should be. But I didn't think that people would be offended, but I was wrong. People were out right upset. After they saw that we weren't changing, they eventually got over it. But my relationships are a little different these days. Food connects people. In America, everything is revolved around food. People love to love food and since we didn't eat the way they did anymore, the connection stopped. I wasn't prepared for this, but again, I made my plan and vision clear. I am dedicated to my mission in becoming my best version and so I continue on.

My husband and I married just after dating for about 10 months. 5 of those months were by phone. We did go to college together and were very good friends, but that didn't prepare us for marriage. When you say hell on earth, it was worse. I just knew I made the wrong decision. But I was committed and dedicated to my marriage. I was committed to not giving up after only a year. And so each and every day we stuck it out. He moved out for a few months. When he came back we probably gave each other the silent treatment for about another few months. We threatened with divorce for a whole year straight but neither one of us could go through with it. I knew it was love there, I just couldn't feel it or see it at that time. You remember when I said I was dedicated to being the person people thought I should be, well that attitude allowed me to have so much baggage going into my marriage that I couldn't even see who the person I was. It took a while for me to figure that out, but when I did my husband and I became partners in life. He is honestly my best friend, I should say my only friend most of the time...lol, but if I was not dedicated to our marriage we would not be where we are now. We wouldn't have created what we now have if it had not been for us being together. He encouraged me to step outside of my comfort zone and when I did, the magic started to happen.

In all that I have said, know that sometimes dedication doesn't mean that you're going to appreciate the change that is going to occur once you make that declaration, make a stance. Nope, it actually means the opposite. You will have to go through some things before you actually see the beauty. When I set out to fix my daughter's scalp issue, it took dedication. When I sought out to heal my body, it took dedication, and as I am building the life I want, it is taking dedication. But once you rise to that peak; peace, joy, happiness, that is when you know, it was all worth it.

Yes, these are my personal stories, but I am sure you all may have some just like mine. Or will experience some like mine, and my advice is to stick with it. You know you are doing it right when it's difficult. Push through it.

>>> If you would like more information on developing your moisture regimen that works for you sign up for our FREE Moisture Regimen Hacking Course at:

www. everbutter.com/MRH

Conclusion

At the end of the day, our decisions will create our life for us. If you seek to go on this journey, there is no other way to have it. Yes, you can make these your truths by tweaking them and making them personal to you, but at the end, if you want healthy hair, the easy way, you have to adopt a lifestyle in order for it to be easy. And that is by taking to heart and adopting the three categories; health, a good regimen, and dedication. Everything in life needs these characteristics. And if you don't, you will drift along being angry at the world because you have not found your best version of yourself.

The saying is that "weeping may endure for the night, but joy comes in the morning". And that is so true. If you are so involved in this standard of living. If you have completely become involved in society, but now you have come to the realization that it hasn't really been working out for you. Get ready for the weeping. But the joy in the morning will feel so good.

Healthy hair is not just about hair. It's about you taking control of who you are. And that control is gone when you have no control over your body. Healthy hair is a healthy body. You cannot have one without the other. If you just want the appearance of health, as so many people love appearances, then everything you seek will be surface level. But if you are looking for the root cause, then your journey has just begun, and I wish you all the best.

>>> If you would like more information on developing your moisture regimen that works for you sign up for our FREE Moisture Regimen Hacking Course at:
www. everbutter.com/MRH

References

Afrika, L., (June 17, 2004), *African Holistic Health*

Fuhrman, J., (October 17, 2017), *Fast Food Genocide*

Moritz, A., (October 1, 2012), *The Amazing Liver and Gallbladder Flush*

Moritz, A., (April 1, 2010), *Heal Yourself with Sunlight*